the ATHL
POCKET GUIDE
to YOGA

50 ROUTINES
for FLEXIBILITY,
BALANCE &
FITNESS

sage rountree

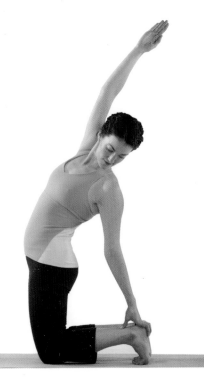

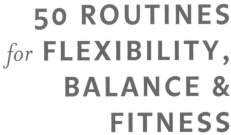

Boulder, Colorado

The Athlete's Pocket Guide to Yoga
Copyright © 2009 by Sage Rountree

▼velopress®

3002 Sterling Circle
Boulder, Colorado 80301-2338 USA

VeloPress is the leading publisher of books on endurance sports. Focused on cycling, triathlon,
running, swimming, and nutrition/diet, VeloPress books help athletes achieve their goals of going
faster and farther. Preview books and contact us at velopress.com.

Distributed in the United States and Canada by Ingram Publisher Services

Library of Congress Cataloging-in-Publication Data
Rountree, Sage Hamilton.
The athlete's pocket guide to yoga / Sage Rountree.
    p. cm.
Includes bibliographical references.
ISBN 978-1-934030-41-7 (pbk.: alk. paper)
1. Hatha yoga. 2. Athletes. I. Title.
RC1220.Y64R684 2009
613.7'046–dc22

                              2009015176

Cover design by Stephanie Goralnick
Cover and interior photos by Don Karle
Interior design by Jane Raese

18 19 20 / 10 9 8 7

CONTENTS

CONTENTS

YOGA *and the* ATHLETE

YOGA AND YOUR TRAINING

Kudos on choosing to begin or deepen your yoga practice! Yoga will enhance your performance as an athlete and make you a better person—not just physically but mentally and spiritually. By practicing yoga, you will develop whole-body strength; increase your flexibility, balance, mental focus, and awareness of your breath; and learn to recognize—and in some cases surpass—the limits of your body.

This book will provide you with shorthand directions for yoga routines appropriate for all phases of your training. I presume that you are familiar with the poses from studying yoga in classes—and perhaps from reading my book *The Athlete's Guide to Yoga: An Integrated Approach to Strength, Flexibility, and Focus* (VeloPress, 2008) and watching the companion DVD, *The Athlete's Guide to Yoga: A Personalized Practice* (Endurance Films, 2008). If you feel unsure about your alignment in a pose, please check with an experienced teacher to be sure you are practicing safely. As you begin any new exercise routine, it's wise to discuss your plans with your health care practitioner.

Yoga in the Training Season
You probably have an annual training plan or a schedule of your athletic season, and your plan probably contains an off-season and base period, a build period in which work is more intense, and a peak or competitive period. Your yoga practice should complement your training, not undermine it, so be sure to keep an inverse relationship between the intensity of your training and the intensity of your yoga practice.

In your off-season and base periods, your training intensity will be light, but you will be focusing on building strength and correcting any imbalances in your body (and you may be using yoga to aid recuperation from an injury). This is the time when your yoga will also focus on strength and on building your range of motion.

As the intensity of your training increases, you'll need to maintain flexibility through yoga. With the exception of core strength poses, your practice should focus on stretching over strengthening. Pay special attention to areas that have been tight in the past, whether that means shoulders, hips, or something else. Be sure that your yoga is enhancing your recovery, not wearing you down. Always err on the side of keeping it mellow.

In your peak and competitive periods, tone down your yoga. *Focus* becomes your focus. You can continue to practice, but choose gentle modifications and restorative poses. Spend some time in meditation each day or every other day.

EQUIPMENT

You don't need much equipment to practice yoga at home. Part of the fun is having a truly personal experience—wearing whatever is on hand, using props with no self-consciousness, setting the mood with music of your choice.

Clothing

Clothing is easy: Wear something comfortable. If you're adding some core strengthening work or hip stretches immediately after a workout, you can probably get away with not changing or even choosing something dirty but dry out of the hamper. In the studio, your classmates appreciate you showing up fragrance-free, but at home, it's not too important. Take care that you do not get a chill by lingering in wet clothing for too long.

Practice in your bare feet. If you are doing a dynamic warm-up or a quick stretch series after a run, running shoes are okay. Avoid practicing in socks—this can be dangerously slippery.

Props

You're practicing at home, in part, to have a highly personalized experience. Don't be shy about using all the props you have available.

A sticky yoga mat is useful but not critical. Floor poses can be done on a rug or carpet; standing poses require a hard surface to provide stability and prevent slipping. If you don't have the space to set a yoga mat on a hard floor, alternate between carpet for floor poses and a hard surface (even if that means a kitchen or bathroom floor) for any poses where only feet or hands are touching the ground. If you're looking to buy, choose a double-thickness, quarter-inch-thick mat and explore eco-friendly options. Prices vary widely: You can buy a thin mat at many stores for under $20 or create a custom design for $85 at Yogamatic.com.

Find something firm to sit on. This can be a yoga bolster, but a folded wool or cotton blanket will work fine, as can a stiff sofa cushion. You can improvise by folding a bed pillow lengthwise and rolling the case, or by stuffing two pillows into one pillowcase. This prop will be useful in seated poses if your hips are tight. You'll sit toward its front edge, so that your knees can release toward the floor. If you're going to splurge on a yoga-specific bolster, look for a rectangular shape, which is more useful than a cylinder. Expect to pay $50 and up for a good bolster.

Blocks make a good prop when the floor seems too far away. You can use them to lengthen your reach toward the floor in standing poses or to prop your knees if they feel lost in space in a pose such as cobbler. Yoga blocks are widely available and cheap (you can find them at many stores for $12 and up), but you can use hardcover books as substitutes. Firmer, heavier blocks provide more stable support than do softer, lighter ones.

A yoga strap is especially useful for athletes. It's critical for the shoulder strap series and hamstring strap series in this book, and it's useful in poses such as cow-face and legs up the wall. A woven yoga strap, which you can get for around $10, is cheap and portable. Be sure to buy a longer strap if you are tall or tight. You might have decent substitutes around the house—a rope, a dog leash, or a tied chain of neckties, belts, or scarves can do.

A kitchen timer or a watch with a countdown timer is another useful prop. This will keep you honest in meditation, and it will help calm some of your restlessness, since you won't be worrying about the time. It can also wake you up should you accidentally fall asleep in corpse pose.

Mood Enhancers
Set the mood for your practice by finding an area free of distractions. This might mean you're in the hallway rather than your home office, or in a guest room instead of the living room.

Perhaps some music is in order. It need not be space music. World beat music is good for yoga, but so is jazz, classical, or anything else you enjoy and don't find distracting. If you've had a busy day, silence may work best.

Remember to turn off your beeping and ringing electronics or move into a space where you can't hear them.

Candles, incense, eye pillows—all of these further set the tone of your choice. And that's the key: It is your space, your time to focus on your body, mind, and breath. Color it however you like.

ALIGNMENT PRINCIPLES

Please study periodically with an experienced teacher of your choice. Having a trained set of eyes on your form is as important in yoga as it is in sports. Follow these guidelines to keep you safe when you practice yoga at home.

Keep Mountain Pose
The alignment of mountain pose—standing tall but relaxed—informs all of the thousands of other poses. Learn mountain pose well and constantly refer back to it as you move into other poses. You will usually be correct if you keep your back and neck long, your chest open, your shoulders low, and your weight balanced evenly on your feet. The following suggestions simply echo instructions for mountain pose.

Check That Knees and Toes Agree
Keep your knees and toes in alignment with each other. When your toes point forward, so should your knees. When your knees point outward, so should your toes. The knee is a hinge joint—don't apply stress to one side of the hinge by setting the knee and toes at odds with each other.

Twist Around a Long Spine
To protect your disks and yield a deeper twist, be sure your spine is always long, never crunched or angled to one side, before you initiate a twist. Propping a hand

on the floor in seated twists can help with this action. In reclining twists, try to keep both shoulders on the floor.

Protect the Neck

In back bends and inversions, don't take the neck too far from its natural curve. When you're upside down in bridge, shoulder stand, or plow, bear most of your weight on your shoulders, not your head.

Work the Safe Side of the Edge

Yoga teaches you to work on an intelligent edge—the point of sustainable intensity. This is something endurance athletes know well. Take each pose no further than a tempo or time trial intensity. Let your poses be deep enough that you can feel the benefit, but never push yourself too far. The frisson of this edge of intensity provides opportunity for growth, but it can also tempt you to go too deeply. Be smart.

As your season progresses or in restorative poses, be sure to tend toward the restful, staying an extra step shy of the threshold experience.

Be Efficient

One goal of your yoga practice—just as in your sport—is to be efficient. Direct energy only where it is truly needed. Don't waste any tension in unnecessary areas. Think of it as a power-saving technique: When you leave a room, turn the lights off. In most poses, you won't need any effort in your face, jaw, or shoulders, so let them relax. See if you can dim the lights in your toes as you stand in balance poses. Direct your energy use to target only the muscles keeping you in alignment in each pose. And don't waste effort in self-judgment, frustration, or mental chatter. Relax your mind and breathe.

BREATHING

You have been breathing since you were born, and you will be breathing until you die. Your breath marks you as alive; similarly, it defines your yoga practice. Take long, slow, deep, nasal breaths for yoga. (If your nose is stuffy, you can breathe through your mouth.) When your attention starts to wander away from what you are doing, direct it back to the breath and you'll be focused in the moment again. Thus, your breath becomes a metaphor for the continuous present moment of your life. It's always here, whether you pay attention or not.

If you catch yourself holding your breath, you may be using too much effort. This often happens in balance and core strength poses. Come back to deep nasal breathing, and you'll find the pose easier to maintain.

If you find yourself gasping, you may have pushed too far. Back off immediately! You should never work to the point of pain. Don't confuse productive intensity with pain on the mat—or in your life.

If you feel nothing, ease a little further into the pose as you exhale. You'll know when you've hit the sweet spot.

If you feel yourself releasing a deep sigh, you're probably in the right place.

HOW TO USE THIS BOOK

This book is intended as a prompt for your home practice. As you continue to work on yoga, you'll learn to follow the lead of your body, and it will become your practice guide. For now, consider the routines in this volume a starting point. Riff on them. Combine them in new ways; try doing the poses in a different order. Play with the modifications and props shown, or devise new versions of the poses. This is how you learn to follow your own path.

Timing in the Day
Where should your yoga fit in the course of your day? It depends.

Warm-ups, restorative poses, breath exercises, and meditation can be done at any time during the day and are especially nice just before a workout or just before bed.

Core poses and deeper stretches for the hips and legs are appropriate immediately after a workout. Be sure you move into them slowly, so that your muscles agree to release for each stretch. When you are going to practice these poses separate from a workout, be sure to add one or two warm-up sequences beforehand.

Some poses have a stimulating nature and are better slotted early in the day or early in a longer practice. These include standing poses, balance poses, most flow routines, and back bends.

Other poses are calming and work well toward the end of a practice or at bedtime. These include the work for the hips and legs, inversions, and the restorative routines outlined in this book.

Your stomach will thank you not to do core work, back bending, or twisting too soon after a meal.

How Long to Hold

Unless otherwise noted, hold each pose for five full breaths. You'll learn in time which poses work well for you when held longer and which have reached maximum efficacy with five or even fewer breaths. Some days you'll need more, some days less.

You'll also get to know your body's imbalances—you may find one hip tighter than the other, or twisting in one direction much freer than twisting in the other. One of the glories of home practice is the ability to linger in a pose, paying attention to exactly what your body needs in the moment. This is especially good for correcting muscular imbalances.

Meditation and Breath Exercises

While meditation and breath exercises appear last in the list of routines, they could have gone first or been included in a separate volume. Since the work of the physical yoga practice is designed to prepare our bodies and minds for meditation, I've slotted meditation and breath work after the poses.

Be comfortable for these exercises. Many teachers warn against lying down for meditation, since it is so conducive to sleep (and this is especially true for tired athletes). If sitting tall on a prop on the floor—knees low, spine long, shoulders relaxed—is too tough, try sitting on a couch or in a comfortable chair. If your back or hips cause you distress that interferes with your concentration, then you can move to the bed or floor and try again there. It's better to pay attention to the practice at hand—and to strengthen your core and open your hips with yoga poses!

Start small in your meditation training. Five minutes is a good beginning point. Try adding a minute or two each session, or even weekly. You'll soon learn how long it takes for your mind to settle down (if it ever does) and for the productive stillness to come in. Build your meditation time slowly, just as you build your mileage. Periodically take a step-back week with reduced volume. Eventually you can meditate for several minutes a few times a week, perhaps with one longer session added on the weekends. One lowball rule of thumb would be to spend x minutes per day in meditation, where x is equal to the number of hours you train per week.

A final word on meditation, yoga, and your training: Each requires a warm-up period, each can be very tough to get into at the beginning, and each benefits from systematic planning and practice. Try logging the time you spend in meditation and on your yoga practice. When your records reveal a consistent practice, you'll be seeing definite results.

Best wishes, and namaste.

YOGA ROUTINES

SPINAL WARM-UP, PRONE
Total time: 5 min.

Dog
Cat
Child's pose
Lateral child's pose
Threading the needle twist

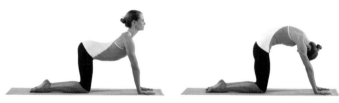

Dog (inhale) and cat (exhale)
10 or more breaths

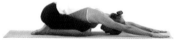

Child's pose
3 breaths

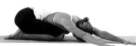

Lateral child's pose
5 breaths per side

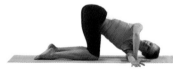

Threading the needle twist
5 breaths per side

TIP ▶ The breath guideline is merely a suggestion;
hold the poses until you feel even side to side.

SPINAL WARM-UP, SUPINE
Total time: 5 min.

Supine lateral stretch
Knees to chest
Hug one knee
Knees-down reclining twist

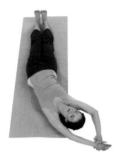 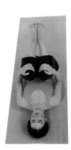 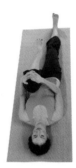

Supine lateral stretch	Knees to chest	Hug one knee
5 breaths per side	5 breaths	5 breaths per side

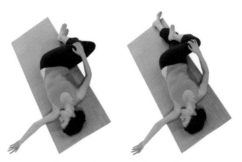

Knees-down reclining twist
5 breaths per side

TIP ▶ For a gentler stretch, let your bottom leg extend down the mat in the reclining twist.

SPINAL WARM-UP, SEATED
Total time: 5 min.

Camel ride
Lateral stretch
Easy twist

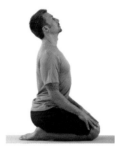 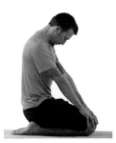

Camel ride
Take dog (inhale) and cat (exhale) from kneeling;
five rounds

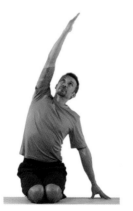 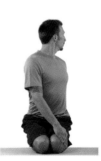

Lateral stretch
Five breaths per side

Easy twist
Five breaths per side

TIP ▸ Sitting on a prop makes these poses feel freer.

HALF SALUTES WITH CHAIR
Total time: 8 min.

Move through three cycles.

Inhale

Salutation

Upward salute

Half forward fold

Upward salute

Exhale

Salutation

Swan dive to forward fold

Full forward fold

Salutation

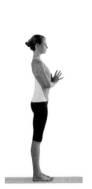

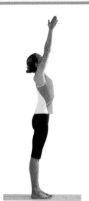

Salutation
Inhale, exhale

Upward salute
Inhale

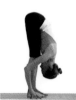

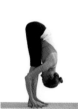

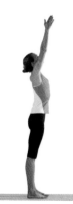

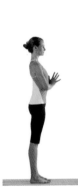

Swan dive to
forward fold
Exhale

Half forward fold
Inhale

Full forward fold
Exhale

Upward salute
Inhale

Salutation
Exhale

(continues)

HALF SALUTES WITH CHAIR
(continued)

Now swap the upward salute for chair and move through three more rounds:

Inhale	**Exhale**
Salutation	*Chair*
Chair	*Swan dive to forward fold*
Half forward fold	*Full forward fold*
Chair	*Salutation*

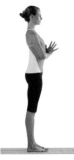 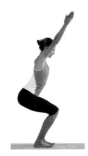

Salutation
Inhale

Chair
Exhale, inhale

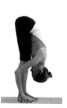 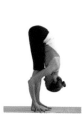 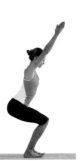 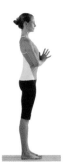

Swan dive to forward fold Exhale	Half forward fold Inhale	Full forward fold Exhale	Chair Inhale	Salutation Exhale

TIP ▸ Practice as many of these cycles as your time and energy allow.

TALL MOUNTAIN FLOW

Total time: 3 min.

Move through the sequence five times.

Balancing toe squat
Roll like a ball
Balancing toe squat
Mountain balance

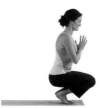

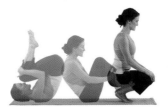

Balancing toe squat
Inhale

Roll like a ball
Exhale back, inhale up

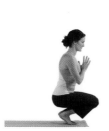

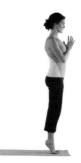

Balancing toe squat
Exhale

Mountain balance
Inhale up, exhale back to squat

TIP ▸ To protect your neck, do not roll back any farther than your shoulders. This sequence is good for finding your center of balance during movement, controlling motion from the core.

CHAIR AND TREE

Total time: 4 min.

Chair
Mountain
Tree
Twisting chair
Tree
Twisting chair
Mountain

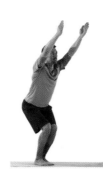

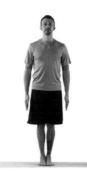

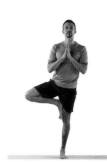

| Chair
5 breaths | Mountain
3 breaths | Tree, right leg bent
5 breaths |

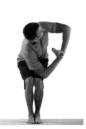

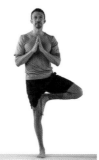

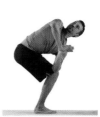

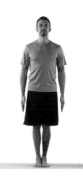

| Twisting chair,
to the left
5 breaths | Tree, left leg bent
5 breaths | Twisting chair,
to the right
5 breaths | Mountain
3 breaths |

TIP ▸ Economize by relaxing your feet as much as you can while staying stable.

STANDING BALANCE FLOW

Total time: 6-8 min.

Move through the sequence below three times, first on one side,
then on the other.

    Flow 1. Hold each pose for five breaths.

    Flow 2. Hold each pose for one breath.

    Flow 3. Move in and out of each pose with the breath.

Dancer
Eagle
Pyramid
Triangle
Half moon

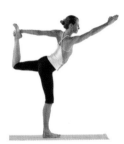 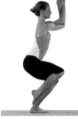 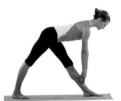

      Dancer   Eagle   Pyramid

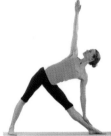 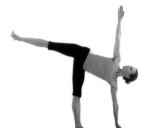

    Triangle   Half moon

TIP ▸ Use your gaze to hold you steady in the postures.
Use a block or move to a wall for half moon if you feel wobbly.

CRANE AND WARRIOR III

Total time: 5-7 min.

Repeat the entire sequence three to five times, holding each pose for a few breaths.

Crane
Forward fold
Upward salute
Warrior III

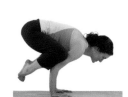 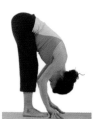

Crane	Forward fold
Inhale	Exhale

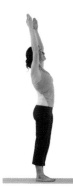 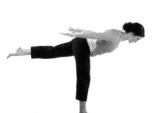 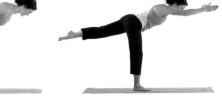

Upward salute	Warrior III
Inhale	Exhale; both sides

TIP ▸ Move very deliberately into the poses; moving too fast will spoil your balance. Choose an arm position that challenges you in warrior III.

SUN SALUTATIONS WITH LUNGES

Total time: 10 min.

Move through the sequence, linking breath and action. Repeat, swapping *right* and *left* sides, to complete one cycle. Complete three to five full cycles using an even breath.

Inhale	Exhale
Salutation	*Salutation*
Upward salute	*Swan dive to forward fold*
Half forward fold	*Full forward fold*
Right leg back to high lunge	*Square hips in lunge*
Arms to knee or overhead	*Fold to ground*
High plank	*Stick*
Upward-facing dog	*Downward-facing dog*
Right leg forward to high lunge	*Square hips in lunge*
Arms to knee or overhead	*Fold to ground*
Left leg forward to the fold	*Full forward fold*
Upward salute	*Salutation*

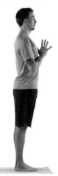

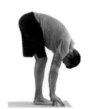
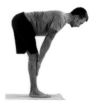

Salutation	Upward salute	Swan dive to forward fold	Half forward fold
Inhale, exhale	Inhale	Exhale	Inhale

(continues)

SUN SALUTATIONS WITH LUNGES
(continued)

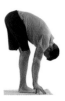

Full forward fold
Exhale

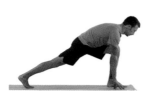

Right leg back to high lunge
Inhale
Square hips in lunge
Exhale

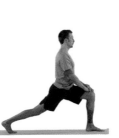

Arms to knee or overhead
Inhale

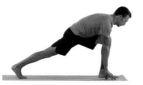

Fold to ground
Exhale

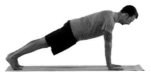

High plank
Inhale

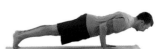

Stick
Exhale

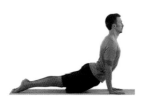

Upward-facing dog
Inhale

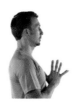

Downward-facing dog
Exhale

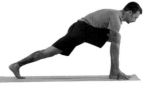

Right leg forward to high lunge
Inhale
Square hips in lunge
Exhale

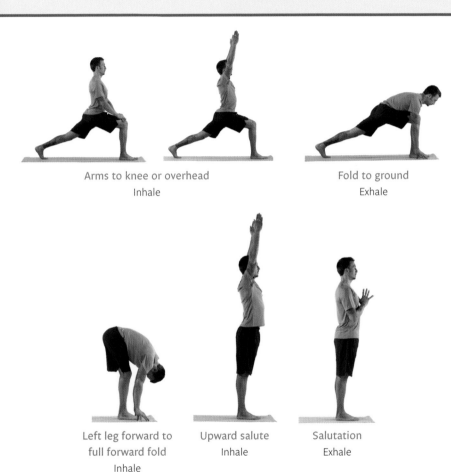

Arms to knee or overhead
Inhale

Fold to ground
Exhale

Left leg forward to
full forward fold
Inhale

Upward salute
Inhale

Salutation
Exhale

TIP ▶ To increase strength and balance in the base period, hold high lunge for three breaths. To improve and maintain hip flexibility as you build training intensity, take a low lunge instead.

23

MOON SALUTATIONS

Total time: 10 min.

Move through the sequence, inhaling as you take the first pose and exhaling as you take the second. Repeat, swapping *right* and *left* sides, to complete one cycle. Aim to complete three full cycles with an even breath.

Inhale	Exhale
Mountain	*Wrist stretch*
Upward salute	*Standing side stretch left*
Upward salute	*Standing side stretch right*
Upward salute	*Wide squat, stepping right*
Star	*Slide to triangle over right leg*
Triangle	*Pyramid, passive back*
Pyramid, active back	*Low lunge*
Crescent lunge	*Hands inside right foot*
Side squat	*Slide across mat*
Side squat	*Low lunge*
Crescent lunge	*Low lunge*
Step in for pyramid, active back	*Fold into pyramid, passive back*
Triangle	*Triangle*
Star	*Squat*
Step right to upward salute	*Standing side stretch left*
Upward salute	*Standing side stretch right*
Upward salute	*Wrist stretch*
Mountain	*Mountain*

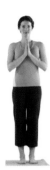

Mountain
Inhale

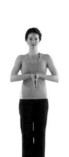

Wrist stretch
Exhale

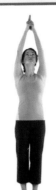

Upward salute
Inhale

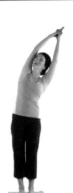

Standing side
stretch left
Exhale

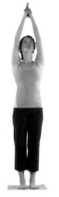

Upward salute
Inhale

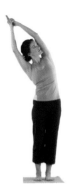

Standing side
stretch right
Exhale

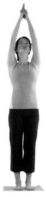

Upward salute
Inhale

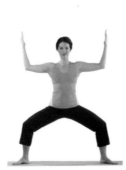

Wide squat,
stepping right
Exhale

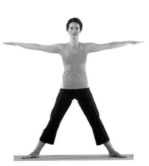

Star
Inhale

(continues)

MOON SALUTATIONS *(continued)*

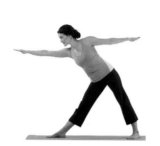

Slide to triangle over right leg
Exhale

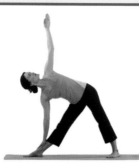

Triangle
Inhale

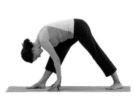

Pyramid, passive back
Exhale

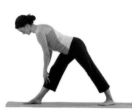

Pyramid, active back
Inhale

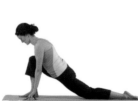

Low lunge
Exhale

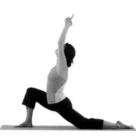

Crescent lunge
Inhale

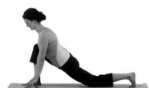

Hands inside right foot
Exhale

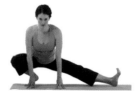

Side squat
Inhale

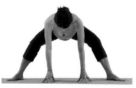

Slide across mat
Exhale

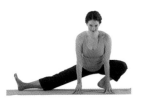

Side squat
Inhale

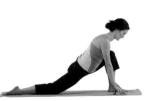

Low lunge
Exhale

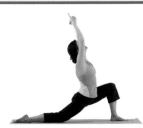

Crescent lunge
Inhale

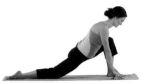

Low lunge
Exhale

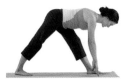

Step in for pyramid,
active back
Inhale

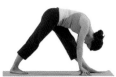

Fold into pyramid,
passive back
Exhale

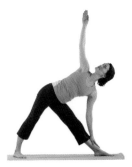

Triangle
Inhale, exhale

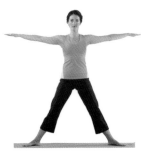

Star
Inhale

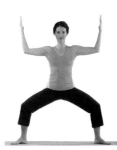

Squat
Exhale

(continues)

MOON SALUTATIONS *(continued)*

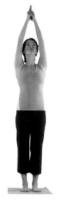

Step right to
upward salute
Inhale

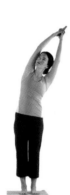

Standing side
stretch left
Exhale

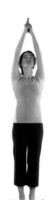

Upward salute
Inhale

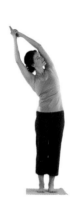

Standing side
stretch right
Exhale

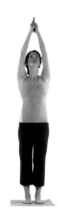

Upward salute
Inhale

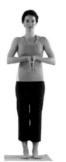

Wrist stretch
Exhale

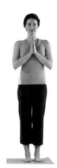

Mountain
Inhale, exhale

TIP ▶ Use the moon salutations to work side to side, as
a complement to the forward motion of your training.

STANDING HIP OPENERS

Total time: 8 min.

Move through the sequence below three times, first on one side,
then on the other.

> Flow 1. Hold each pose for five breaths.
> Flow 2. Hold each pose for one breath.
> Flow 3. Move in and out of each pose with the breath.

Triangle
Side angle
Warrior II
Exalted warrior

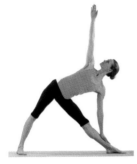

Triangle

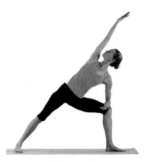

Side angle

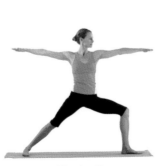

Warrior II

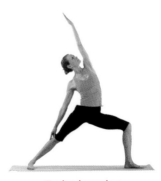

Exalted warrior

TIP ▶ Keep the pinkie-toe side of each foot in contact
with the floor to prevent collapsing into the arch.

STATIC CORE
Total time: 8 min.

Begin by holding each of the poses for three to five breaths; build to ten over time.

Plank
Side plank
Reverse table/reverse plank
Boat

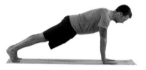 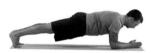

Plank
On palms or forearms

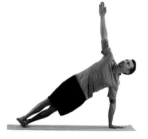 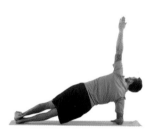

Side plank
On palms or forearms; both sides

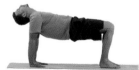 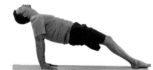 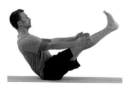

Reverse table or reverse plank

Boat

TIP ▶ Remember mountain alignment in each pose.

DYNAMIC CORE
Total time: 8 min.

Flow through the sequence five to seven times.

Inhale	**Exhale**
Staff	*Roll down to back*
Lift legs over hips	*Plow*
Raise legs over hips	*Lower legs to floor*
Roll up to staff	*Seated forward fold*

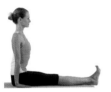

Staff

Inhale

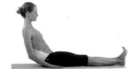

Roll down to back

Exhale

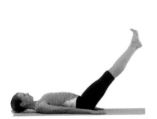

Lift legs over hips

Inhale

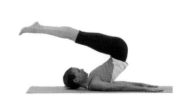

Plow

Exhale

(continues)

DYNAMIC CORE *(continued)*

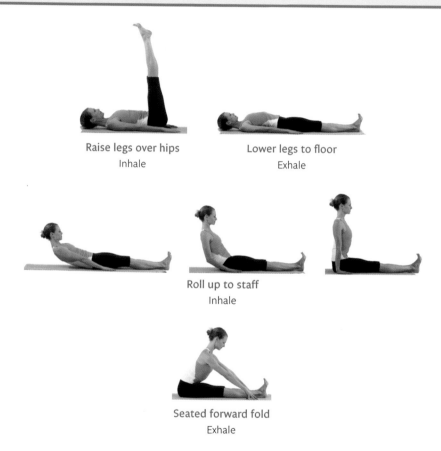

Raise legs over hips
Inhale

Lower legs to floor
Exhale

Roll up to staff
Inhale

Seated forward fold
Exhale

TIP ▸ To make the first part of the sequence easier, bend your knees.
For an added challenge, work with your legs straight and your arms overhead.

Then inhale to staff, exhale and roll down to back. Inhale to lift legs, exhale.

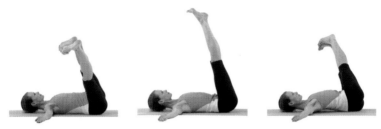

Reclining twists
Lower legs (inhale), raise to midline (exhale); 5 to 7 times

Inhale to bridge, exhale.

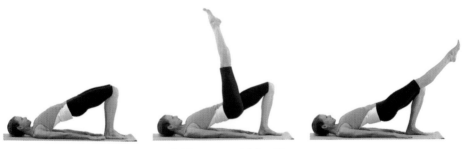

Bridge pose with leg lifts
Lift leg (inhale), lower midway (exhale); 5 to 7 lifts, then switch sides

As you twist, bending and separating the knees will lighten any strain; straight legs will mean more intensity.

TABLE CORE SEQUENCE
Total time: 10 min.

Work both sides in each posture before moving to the next pose.
Aim for at least five breaths in each pose.

Bird dog
Crossbow
Modified side plank
Half moon balance on knee
Side bow

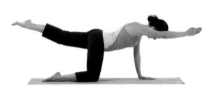

Bird dog
Both sides

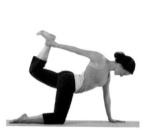

Crossbow
Both sides

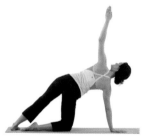

Modified side plank
Both sides

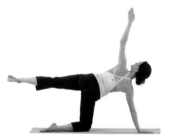

Half moon balance on knee
Both sides

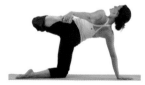

Side bow
Both sides

TIP ▸ Take a rest in child's pose as needed.

CAMEL

Total time: 4-6 min.

Hold each pose for at least five breaths.

Lateral camel stretch
Child's pose
Camel
Child's pose
Camel
Rabbit

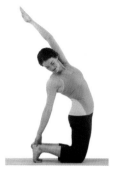

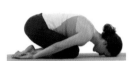

Lateral camel stretch
Both sides

Child's pose

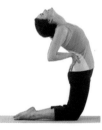

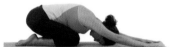

Camel
Hands to sacrum

Child's pose
Arms extended

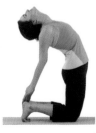

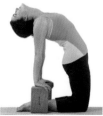

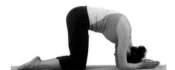

Camel
Hands to blocks or heels

Rabbit

TIP ▶ Keep your hips forward in camel, with a slight tuck of the tailbone. This protects your lower back and further opens the front of the body.

BOW SEQUENCE
Total time: 4 min.

Hold each pose for three to five breaths.

Half bow
Bow
Upward-facing bow

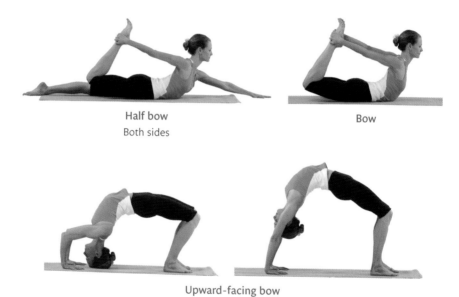

Half bow
Both sides

Bow

Upward-facing bow

TIP ▸ Rest on your belly or back as needed. As you progress,
repeat each move in the sequence three times.

SUPPORTED BACK BENDS
Total time: 6 min.

Hold each pose for eight to ten breaths.
Use a bolster, blanket, or folded pillow as your prop.

Reclining cobbler
Supported fish
Reclining hero

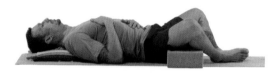

Reclining cobbler

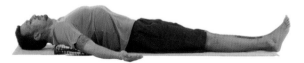

Supported fish

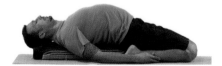

Reclining hero

TIP ▶ These poses are especially useful after a bike workout.

SHOULDER STRAP SERIES

Total time: 5 min.

Shoulder strap circles
Biceps stretch
Triceps stretch

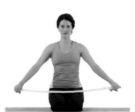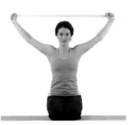

Shoulder strap circles, inhaling to sticking point overhead
Inhale up, exhale down; five times

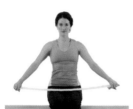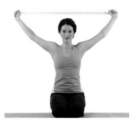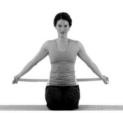

Shoulder strap circles, loosening grip and lowering arms behind back
Inhale up, exhale down; five times

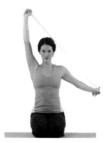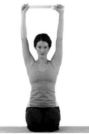

Biceps stretch
Five breaths per side

Triceps stretch
Inhale up, exhale down; five times

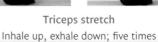

TIP ▶ Keep your shoulder blades low on your back throughout.

INTERLACED FINGERS SERIES
Total time: 4 min.

Hold each pose for at least five breaths.

Fingers in front
Fingers overhead
Side stretch
Fingers behind back
Hands to side waist

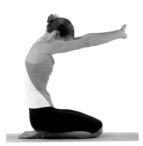

Fingers in front, cat back

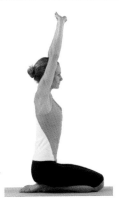

Fingers overhead,
palms up

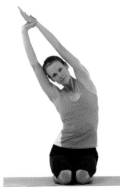

Side stretch
Both sides

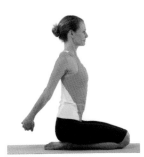

Fingers behind back

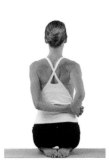

Hands to side waist
Both sides

TIP ▸ Perform these stretches sitting, kneeling, or standing.
Turn your head in the last pose to find the best neck stretch for your body.

WALL SHOULDER STRETCHES
Total time: 5 min.

Hold each pose for at least five breaths.

Push the wall
Clock-face stretch

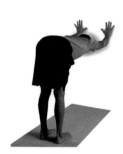

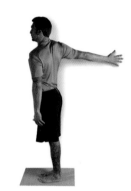

Push the wall

Clock-face stretch, three o'clock
Both sides

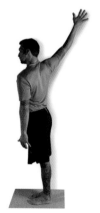

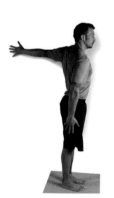

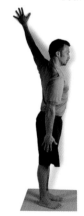

Clock-face stretch,
one o'clock
Both sides

Clock-face stretch,
nine o'clock
Both sides

Clock-face stretch,
eleven o'clock
Both sides

TIP ▸ Experiment with different arm positions
to find an individually appropriate stretch.

40

LUNGE SERIES

Total time: 10 min.

Move through the sequence first on one side, then the other, holding each pose for at least five breaths.

Low lunge
Balancing low lunge
Crescent lunge
Quadriceps stretch in lunge
Prayer twist from lunge
Groin stretch from lunge
Runner's lunge

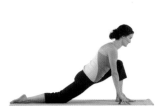

Low lunge

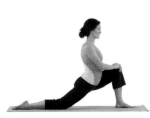

Balancing low lunge

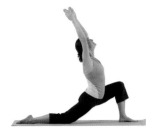

Crescent lunge

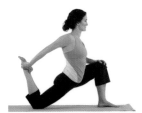

Quadriceps stretch in lunge

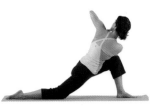

Prayer twist from lunge

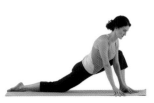

Groin stretch from lunge

(continues)

LUNGE SERIES *(continued)*

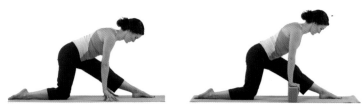

Runner's lunge, toes down

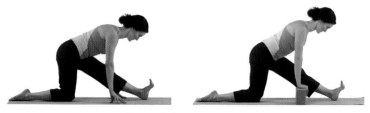

Runner's lunge, toes up

TIP ▸ Keep your hips level and square throughout, and make sure your knees and toes face the same direction.

BOWING SEQUENCES

Total time: 8 min.

Move through the poses, alternately folding over the right leg and the left leg.

Rishi fold
Pyramid

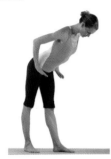

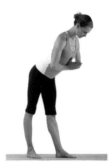

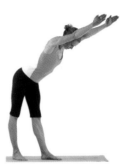

Rishi fold,
hands to hips

Rishi fold, hands in
prayer position

Rishi fold,
arms extended

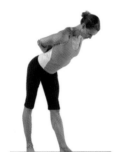

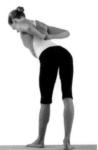

Rishi fold, hands holding elbows
or in reverse prayer

(continues)

BOWING SEQUENCES *(continued)*

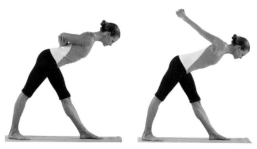

Pyramid, fingers holding elbows
or interlaced behind back

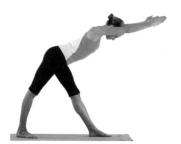

Pyramid, arms extended

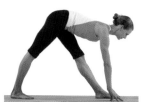

Pyramid, hands reaching
to frame front foot

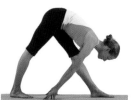

Pyramid, hands toward
back foot

TIP ▸ Bend the knees slightly to keep the hamstrings safe.
Experiment with these different arm positions to find a
good chest stretch that also challenges your core.

PIGEON SERIES

Total time: 10 min.

Repeat the sequence on both sides from dog/cat.

Ball squat
Dog/cat
Pigeon forward fold
Pigeon back bend
Head to knee
Revolved head to knee

Ball squat

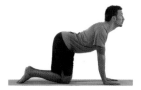

Dog
Inhale

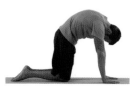

Cat
Exhale

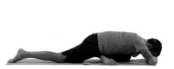

Pigeon forward fold
Ten or more breaths

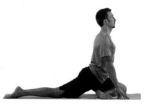

Pigeon back bend
Five or more breaths

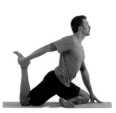

**Pigeon back bend
with optional
quad stretch**
Five or more breaths

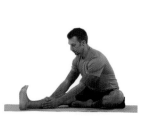

Head to knee
Five or more breaths

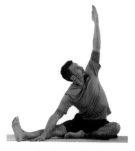

Revolved head to knee
Five or more breaths

TIP ▸ If you feel knee pain in pigeon,
drop to the hip of the forward leg.

45

HEAD TO KNEE SEQUENCE

Total time: 6-8 min.

Perform the sequence on one side, then the other.
Hold each pose at least five breaths.

Head to knee
Revolved head to knee
Sage twist

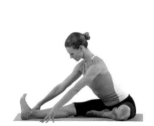 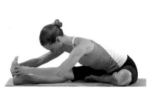

Head to knee

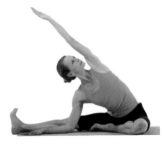

Revolved head to knee

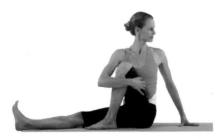 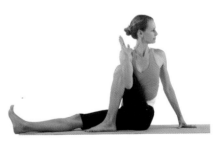

Sage twist

TIP ▸ The head to knee poses help release the quadratus lumborum—
you'll feel the stretch in your back, just above the waistline, on the
side with the leg bent.

IT BAND FLOW
Total time: 8 min.

Hold each pose—except transitions—for at least five breaths.

Cow-face fold
Half Lord of the Fishes
High lunge with groin stretch
Standing spread-legged forward fold; twist
High lunge with groin stretch
Cow-face fold
Half Lord of the Fishes

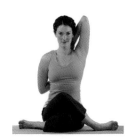
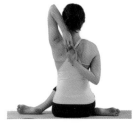
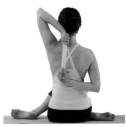

Cow-face fold, right leg on top

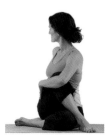
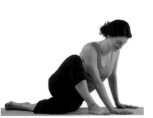
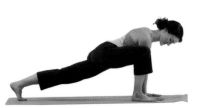

Half Lord of
the Fishes,
right leg on top

Rotate counterclockwise

High lunge with groin stretch

(continues)

IT BAND FLOW *(continued)*

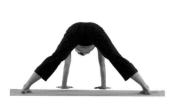

Standing spread-legged
forward fold

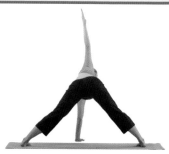

Standing spread-legged forward
fold, twisting left, then right

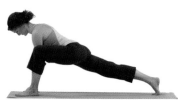

High lunge with groin stretch

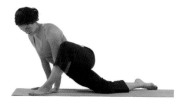

Transition to cow-face legs

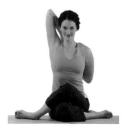

Cow-face fold,
left leg on top

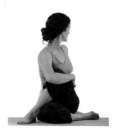

Half Lord of the Fishes,
left leg on top

TIP ▸ Transition to the standing spread-legged forward fold
by spinning on the balls of your feet.

HAMSTRING STRAP SERIES

Total time: 12 min.

Move through the strap series outlined below, spending at least five breaths in each stretch. Start with the left leg bent and the strap on the ball of the right foot, and move through the sequence before repeating on the second side.

Calf stretch
Hamstring stretch
Hamstring stretch with crunch
Deeper hamstring stretch
Outer hamstring stretch
Inner hamstring stretch
Inner thigh stretch
Outer thigh stretch

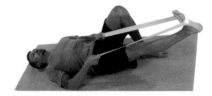

Calf stretch

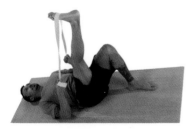

Hamstring stretch

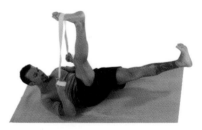

Hamstring stretch with crunch
Engage abs (exhale), extend right leg (inhale);
return head to floor

(continues)

HAMSTRING STRAP SERIES *(continued)*

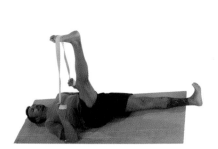

Deeper hamstring stretch

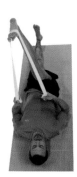

Outer hamstring
stretch

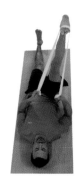

Inner hamstring
stretch

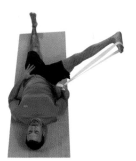

Inner thigh stretch

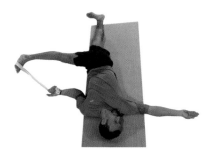

Outer thigh stretch

TIP ▶ Bend your knee as needed to fine-tune the stretches.

SYMMETRICAL STRETCHES
Total time: 4 min.

Hold each pose for at least five breaths.

Wide-angle fold
Cobbler
Star
Frog-legged IT band stretch
Seated forward fold

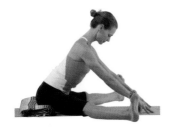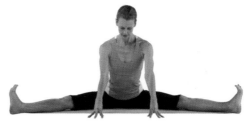

Wide-angle fold

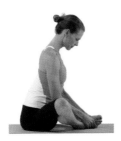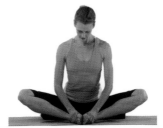

Cobbler

(continues)

SYMMETRICAL STRETCHES *(continued)*

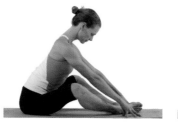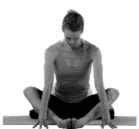

Star

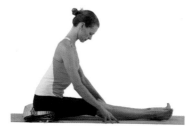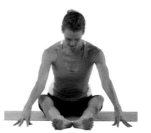

Frog-legged IT band stretch

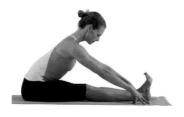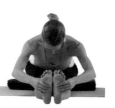

Seated forward fold

TIP ▸ Sit on a folded blanket to make the poses more comfortable.

LOWER-LEG STRETCHES
Total time: 5 min.

Repeat on both sides.

Kneeling Achilles stretch
Front ankle stretch
Toe stretch
Figure 4 with finger/toe stretch

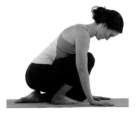 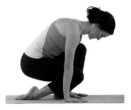

Kneeling Achilles stretch   **Front ankle stretch**

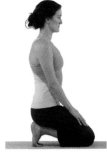 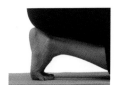

Toe stretch

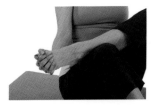 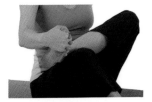

Figure 4 with finger/toe stretch
Point and flex the foot

TIP ▶ Try warming up the legs for these stretches
with a few one-legged balance poses.

GENTLE STRETCHES

Total time: 10 min.

Hold each pose for at least five breaths.

Push the wall
Clock-face stretch
Wide squat
Tight squat
Kneeling
Rishi twist
Seated forward fold
Shoulder stand

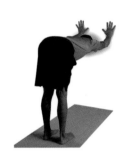

Push the wall

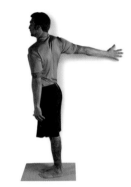

Clock-face stretch, three o'clock
Both sides

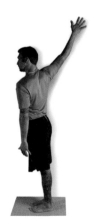

Clock-face stretch,
one o'clock
Both sides

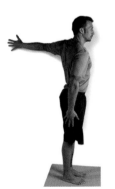

Clock-face stretch,
nine o'clock
Both sides

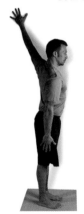

Clock-face stretch,
eleven o'clock
Both sides

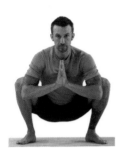

Wide squat

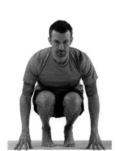

Tight squat

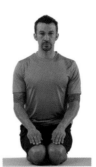

Kneeling

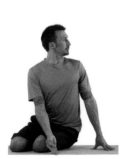

Rishi twist
Both sides

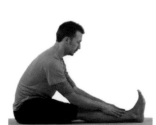

Seated forward fold

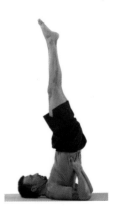

Shoulder stand

TIP ▶ Try unwinding before bed with this sequence.

55

WALL FOLDS

Total time: 6-8 min.

Stay in each pose for at least five breaths.

Wide-angle fold at the wall
Cobbler at the wall
Figure 4 at the wall
Legs up the wall

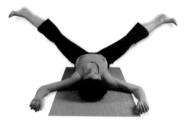

Wide-angle fold at the wall

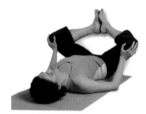

Cobbler at the wall

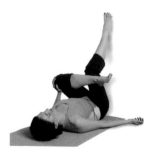

Figure 4 at the wall
Both sides

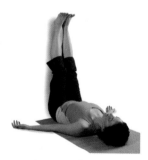

Legs up the wall

TIP ▸ If you find forward folds especially challenging, practicing from this perspective can help build flexibility while keeping your back in neutral alignment.

INVERSIONS
Total time: 5 min.

Try to hold each inversion for ten breaths.

Half shoulder stand
Shoulder stand
Plow
Snail
Fish
Happy baby

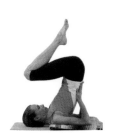
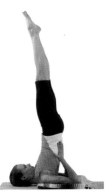

Half shoulder stand   Shoulder stand

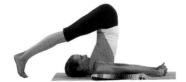
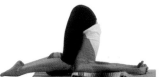

Plow   Snail

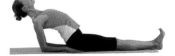
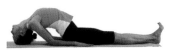
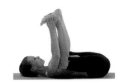

Fish
Five breaths

Happy baby

TIP ▸ While these poses are great after a long workout
or race, don't invert too soon after a hard effort, or
you may become nauseated.

RECLINING TWISTS

Total time: 8 min.

Run through the entire sequence on one side before moving to the other.
Hold each pose for at least five breaths.

Figure 4
Reclining Half Lord of the Fishes
Cross-legged reclining twist

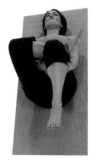 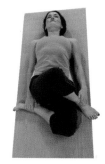

Figure 4   Reclining Half Lord
of the Fishes

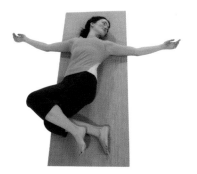 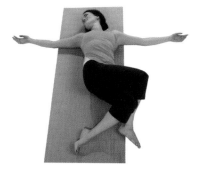

Cross-legged reclining twist
Both ways

TIP ▸ Keep your shoulder girdle level
against the floor throughout.

SUPPORTED STRETCHES
Total time: 20+ min.

Use a bolster, rolled blanket, or folded bed pillow as your prop.

Child's pose
Seated forward fold
Squatting
Supported fish
Knees-down prone twist
Shoulder stand

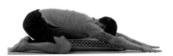

Child's pose, belly to bolster

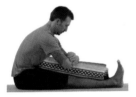
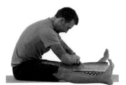
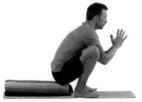

Seated forward fold,
bolster on or between thighs

Squatting on bolster

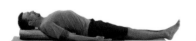
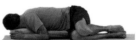
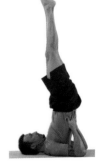

Supported fish on bolster

Knees-down prone twist,
belly to bolster
Both sides

Shoulder stand

TIP ▸ Choose or create a bolster big enough
to make you feel completely supported.

CORPSE POSE

Total time: 3+ min.

Corpse pose

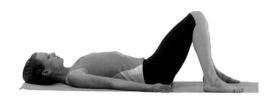

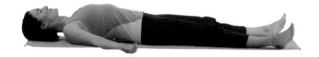

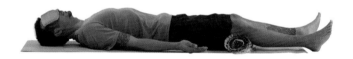

Half corpse, corpse, or corpse with props
Easy, natural breathing

TIP ▸ Add this after each yoga session,
no matter how busy you feel.

CENTERING
Total time: 3+ min.

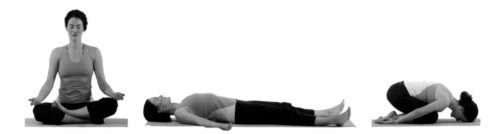

Get comfortable, either seated, resting on your back, or in child's pose.

Run through the inventory of your senses as you turn your attention inward: Notice the quality of the light filtered through your shut eyes. Hear the sounds in the room. Smell the air as it enters through your nostrils. Toward the end of an exhalation, swallow and notice any ambient taste. Feel the points of your body in contact with the air, the floor, and your clothing.

Then turn your awareness exclusively to your breath, perhaps inserting one of the breath exercises here.

Set an intention before you move on.

TIP ▶ You can move through this meditation exercise many times over the course of a session or a day.

THE BREATH IN SPACE
Total time: 7 min.

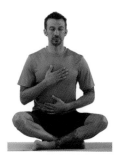
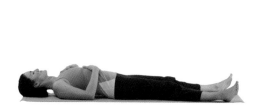

Seated or reclining, with one hand on your belly and the other on your chest, engage a full, deep breath. Spend five to ten breaths moving your breath through each of the following patterns:

Belly, rib cage, upper chest (inhale); upper chest, rib cage, belly (exhale)
Upper chest, rib cage, belly (inhale); belly, rib cage, upper chest (exhale)
Rib cage, then upper chest and belly (inhale and exhale)
All three areas at once (inhale and exhale)

Finish with a few natural breaths.

TIP ▶ Once you are familiar with the muscles of respiration, try the same sequence with your hands in your lap.

THE BREATH IN TIME

Total time: 5 min.

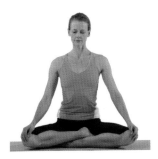

Be comfortable, seated or reclining, and bring your awareness to your breath. First notice its natural rhythm. Then bring the inhalation and exhalation to equal duration, counting each to eight or so (pace this however it feels natural).

Next play with these variations.

Inhale 8, exhale 10
Inhale 8, rest in fullness 2, exhale 8, rest in emptiness 2
Inhale 8, rest in fullness 2, exhale 10, rest in emptiness 2

Return to natural breathing for a few rounds as needed between exercises and to finish.

TIP ▸ Breath ratio exercises are especially useful for swimmers.

ALTERNATE-NOSTRIL BREATHING

Total time: 3 min.

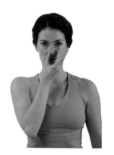 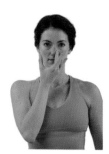

Take a comfortable seat and bring the middle fingers of the right hand and the right thumb to your nose. Inhale through the left nostril, exhale through the right nostril. Inhale through the right nostril, exhale through the left nostril.

Repeat for a total of five or more cycles.

TIP ► Whether or not you feel the subtle energy balancing effected by this exercise, enjoy the focus it yields and notice how it quiets the mind.

COUNTING MEDITATION

Total time: 5+ min.

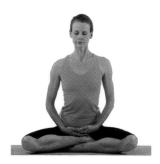

From a comfortable seat, eyes half open or closed, bring your attention to your breath. Breathing in, count to yourself, *thirty*, and breathing out, count *twenty-nine*. Continue until you find that you have lost focus; resume counting from thirty. If you get to zero, simply sit for the predetermined time.

TIP ▶ Set your watch or a timer to keep you on track.

OBSERVATION MEDITATION

Total time: 5+ min.

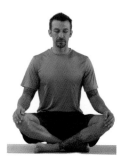

Get comfortable. Lower your gaze or shut your eyes. Bring your attention to your breathing and observe what happens. When your attention wanders, notice what's happening and bring your awareness back to the breath. Don't slip into self-judgment—it's perfectly natural for the mind to go off-track. The work is in mindfully directing yourself away from chattering thoughts and back to the breath.

When your allotted time is up, take a few deep breaths to gradually direct your attention outward.

TIP ▸ Resist the urge to cut your session short when you butt up against discomfort, either physical or mental. Abide. Observe what is happening without intervening and return to breath awareness. This is the real work of meditation.

CLOSING
Total time: 3 min.

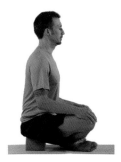

Find a comfortable seated postion, perhaps on a prop. Over the course of a few breaths, notice the state of your body, mind, and spirit. Return to the intention you set as you began your practice. Resist any impulse to judge; simply realign with your sense of purpose. You might form a new intention to take with you off the mat.

Take a moment to offer gratitude, devotion, or dedication of your practice in a way that feels right for you.

Finish with your hands at your heart, and bow to the divine in you and in everyone. Namaste.

TIP ▸ Move very slowly at the end of your practice, so you can take the good feeling with you.

part 3

FOCUSED ROUTINES *and*
COMBINING SEQUENCES

GETTING STARTED

The routines listed in Part 2 can be combined into your own practice sequences. How you combine the routines will depend on where you are in your season. Remember, your yoga practice should complement and support your training. This usually means the physical stress of the yoga should be in inverse proportion to the amount of work you are doing in your other modalities. The routines listed here focus on strength, power, flexibility, and restoration.

Trying these combinations of the routines will give you templates with which you can begin creating your own sessions. As your practice deepens, you will get a feel for what poses are appropriate at any given point both in the session and in the season. Personalizing your practice allows room for spontaneity and lets you address your individual needs. Just as in training, progress comes when you focus on the work you find challenging instead of simply playing up your strengths.

In general, for a longer practice you should include some centering, possibly with a breath exercise; a warm-up; a sequence of standing or balance poses; work for the core, including the back; and floor work with stretches for the legs, twists for the spine, and inversions to calm the nervous system. A shorter practice might follow a workout and include simply standing poses, just core, exclusively hip stretches—or a combination of these. Or you might focus on the more subtle breath exercises and meditation.

However long your practice, don't shortchange yourself by skipping corpse pose, which begins your integration of the practice. Remember, we grow stronger from training not during the workouts, which stress the body, but during recovery, as the body integrates the work and anticipates more work to come. Even one minute spent resting and breathing in corpse pose after a ten-minute home practice yields benefits.

FOCUS ON STRENGTH

A more powerful, strength-based practice is appropriate during your off-season and base periods.

To create a long routine, start with centering, breath work, then a warm-up; proceed into standing poses and balance work; move to core work and back bends; then finish with stretches for the hips and legs, inversions and twists, and corpse pose. Here are three hour-long routines that follow this model.

Strength Routine 1 (1 hr.)

Centering
The breath in space
Half salutes with chair
Sun salutations with lunges
Standing balance flow
Static core
Bow sequence
Symmetrical stretches
Inversions
Corpse pose
Closing

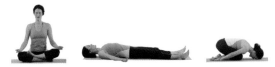

CENTERING
> p. 61

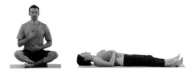

THE BREATH IN SPACE
> p. 62

(continues)

Strength Routine 1 (continued)

HALF SALUTES WITH CHAIR
> pp. 15–16

SUN SALUTATIONS WITH LUNGES
> pp. 21–23

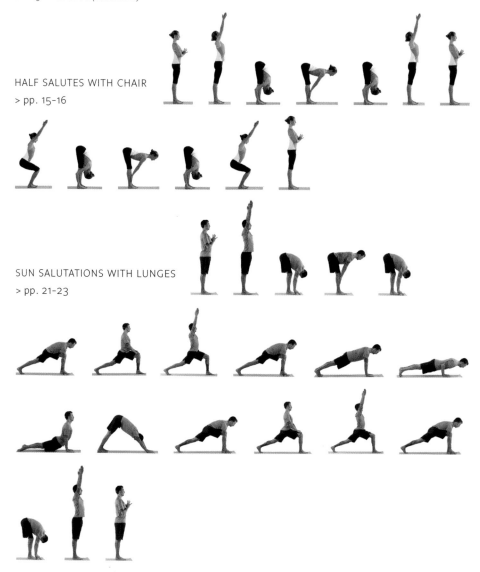

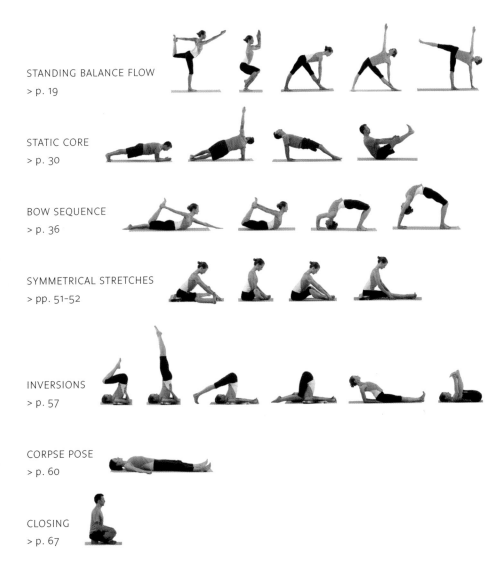

STANDING BALANCE FLOW
> p. 19

STATIC CORE
> p. 30

BOW SEQUENCE
> p. 36

SYMMETRICAL STRETCHES
> pp. 51–52

INVERSIONS
> p. 57

CORPSE POSE
> p. 60

CLOSING
> p. 67

Strength Routine 2 (1 hr.)

Centering
The breath in time
Spinal warm-up, supine
Tall mountain flow
Standing hip openers
Dynamic core
Camel pose
Lunge series
Reclining twists
Corpse pose
Closing

CENTERING
> p. 61

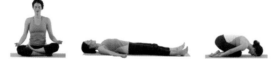

THE BREATH IN TIME
> p. 63

SPINAL WARM-UP, SUPINE
> p. 13

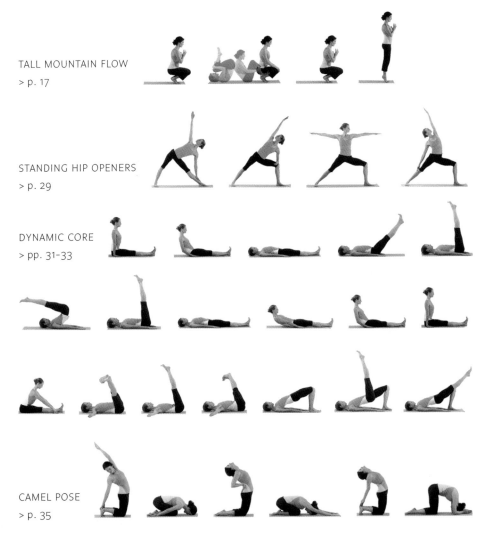

TALL MOUNTAIN FLOW
> p. 17

STANDING HIP OPENERS
> p. 29

DYNAMIC CORE
> pp. 31–33

CAMEL POSE
> p. 35

(continues)

Strength Routine 2 (continued)

LUNGE SERIES
> pp. 41-42

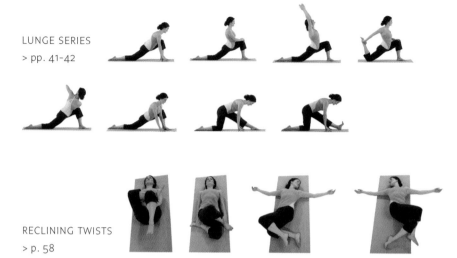

RECLINING TWISTS
> p. 58

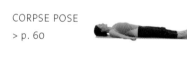

CORPSE POSE
> p. 60

CLOSING
> p. 67

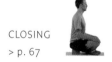

Strength Routine 3 (1 hr.)

Centering
Alternate-nostril breathing
Spinal warm-up, seated
Chair and tree
Crane and warrior III
Table core sequence
Bowing sequences
Gentle stretches
Corpse pose
Closing

CENTERING
> p. 61

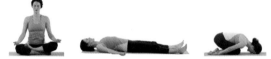

ALTERNATE-NOSTRIL BREATHING
> p. 64

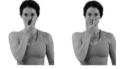

SPINAL WARM-UP, SEATED
> p. 14

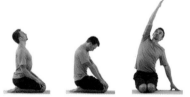

(continues)

Strength Routine 3 (continued)

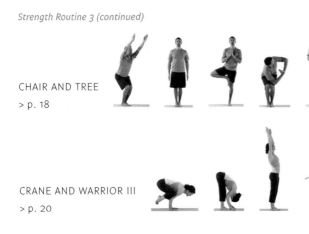

CHAIR AND TREE

> p. 18

CRANE AND WARRIOR III

> p. 20

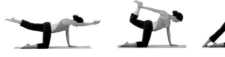

TABLE CORE SEQUENCE

> p. 34

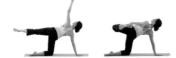

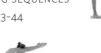

BOWING SEQUENCES

> pp. 43-44

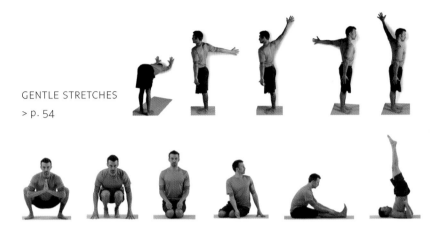

GENTLE STRETCHES
> p. 54

CORPSE POSE
> p. 60

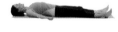

CLOSING
> p. 67

FOCUS ON POWER

Shorter, power-based routines could include a dynamic warm-up (this could even be slotted before your workout). Follow with balance, core work, and back bends, then move to flexibility training as time allows or your personal imbalances require. Here are some twenty-minute combinations to try.

Power-Based Routine 1 (20 min.)

Half salutes with chair
Dynamic core
Camel pose
IT band flow

HALF SALUTES WITH CHAIR
> pp. 15–16

DYNAMIC CORE
> pp. 31–33

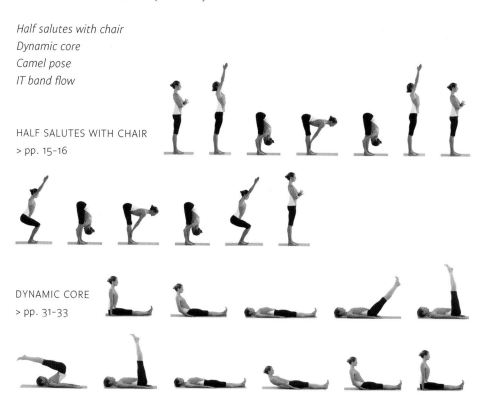

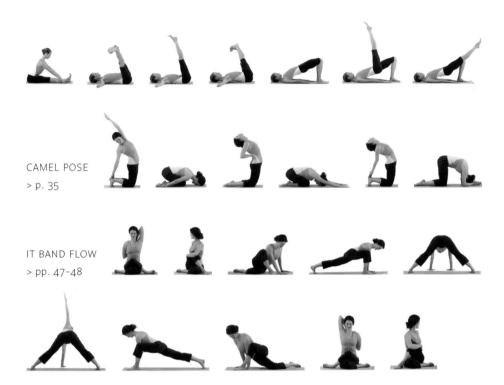

CAMEL POSE
> p. 35

IT BAND FLOW
> pp. 47-48

Power-Based Routine 2 (20 min.)

Sun salutations with lunges
Static core
Bow sequence
Bowing sequences

SUN SALUTATIONS WITH LUNGES
> pp. 21–23

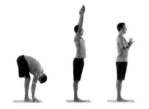

STATIC CORE
> p. 30

BOW SEQUENCE
> p. 36

BOWING SEQUENCES
> pp. 43-44

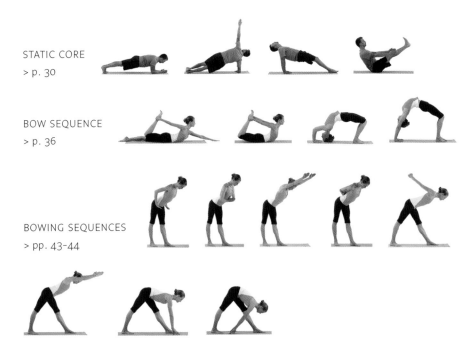

Power-Based Routine 3 (20 min.)

Tall mountain flow
Table core sequence
Head to knee sequence

TALL MOUNTAIN FLOW
> p. 17

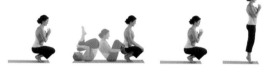

TABLE CORE SEQUENCE
> p. 34

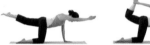

HEAD TO KNEE SEQUENCE
> p. 46

FOCUS ON FLEXIBILITY

As your training intensifies, your practice should help you stay loose. Full routines can include the standing work that is appropriate in the base period, but go for shorter holds or fewer repetitions of the poses. Target your efforts toward stretching the shoulders, hips, and legs, and be sure to address whatever sport-specific needs you have.

Hour-long routines might include the following.

Flexibility Routine 1 (1 hr.)

Centering
The breath in space
Spinal warm-up, prone
Half salutes with chair
Standing hip openers
Shoulder strap series
Lunge series
Lower-leg stretches
Wall folds
Corpse pose
Closing

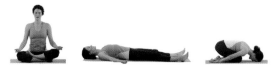

CENTERING
> p. 61

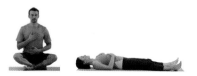

THE BREATH IN SPACE
> p. 62

(continues)

Flexibility Routine 1 (continued)

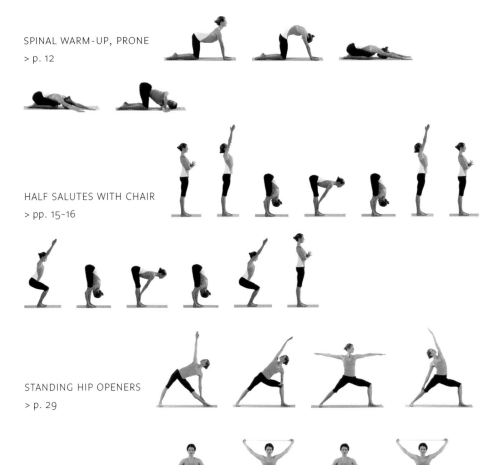

SPINAL WARM-UP, PRONE
> p. 12

HALF SALUTES WITH CHAIR
> pp. 15–16

STANDING HIP OPENERS
> p. 29

SHOULDER STRAP SERIES
> p. 38

LUNGE SERIES
> pp. 41-42

LOWER-LEG STRETCHES
> p. 53

  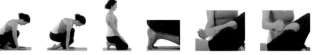

WALL FOLDS
> p. 56

CORPSE POSE
> p. 60

CLOSING
> p. 67

87

FOCUSED ROUTINES *and* COMBINING SEQUENCES

Flexibility Routine 2 (1 hr.)

Centering
The breath in time
Spinal warm-up, supine
Moon salutations
Interlaced fingers series
Head to knee sequence
Hamstring strap series
Inversions
Corpse pose
Closing

 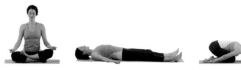

CENTERING
> p. 61

THE BREATH IN TIME
> p. 63

SPINAL WARM-UP, SUPINE
> p. 13

88

MOON SALUTATIONS
> pp. 24-28

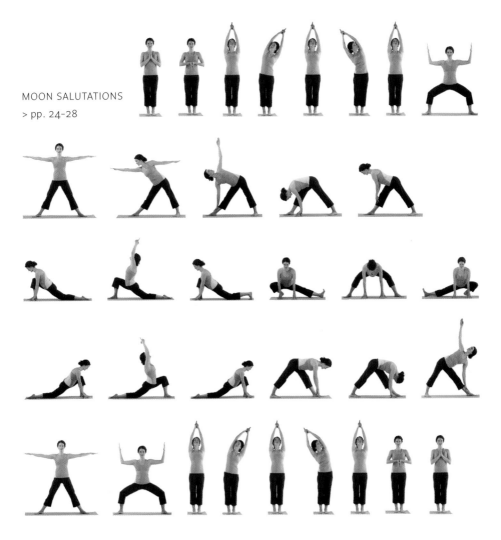

(continues)

Flexibility Routine 2 (continued)

INTERLACED FINGERS SERIES
> p. 39

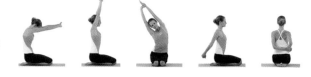

HEAD TO KNEE SEQUENCE
> p. 46

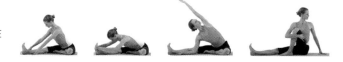

HAMSTRING STRAP SERIES
> pp. 49–50

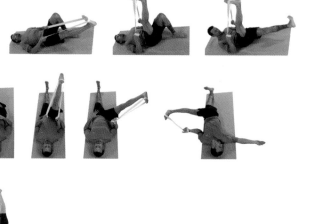

INVERSIONS
> p. 57

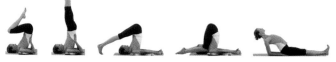

CORPSE POSE
> p. 60

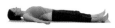

CLOSING
> p. 67

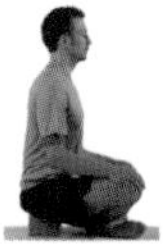

Flexibility Routine 3 (1 hr.)

Centering
Alternate-nostril breathing
Spinal warm-up, seated
Tall mountain flow
Bowing sequences
IT band flow
Gentle stretches
Corpse pose
Closing

CENTERING
> p. 61

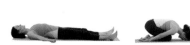

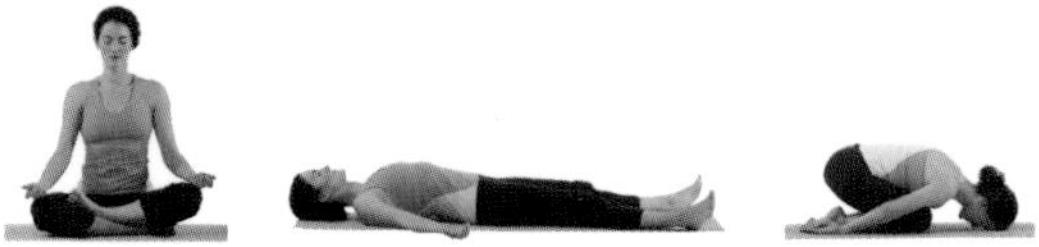

ALTERNATE-NOSTRIL BREATHING
> p. 64

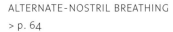
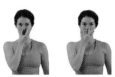

(continues)

Flexibility Routine 3 (continued)

SPINAL WARM-UP, SEATED
> p. 14

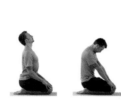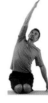

TALL MOUNTAIN FLOW
> p. 17

BOWING SEQUENCES
> pp. 43-44

IT BAND FLOW
> pp. 47-48

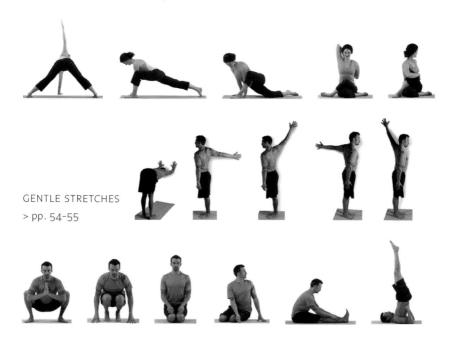

GENTLE STRETCHES
> pp. 54-55

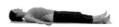

CORPSE POSE
> p. 60

CLOSING
> p. 67

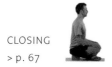

Shorter Flexibility Routines

These can be added immediately following your workouts. Here are some
examples, each lasting about twenty minutes.

After a Swim, Climb, or Ball Game (20 min.)

Interlaced-fingers series
Symmetrical stretches
Gentle stretches

INTERLACED FINGERS SERIES
> p. 39

SYMMETRICAL STRETCHES
> pp. 51-52

GENTLE STRETCHES
> pp. 54-55

After a Ride (20 min.)

Supported back bends
Lunge series
Reclining twists

SUPPORTED BACK BENDS
> p. 37

LUNGE SERIES
> pp. 41–42

RECLINING TWISTS
> p. 58

After a Run or Cross-Country Skiing (20 min.)

Pigeon series
Lower-leg stretches
or
Hamstring strap series
Reclining twists

PIGEON SERIES
> p. 45

LOWER-LEG STRETCHES
> p. 53

or

HAMSTRING STRAP SERIES
> pp. 49–50

  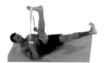

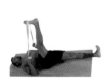   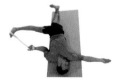

RECLINING TWISTS
> p. 58

FOCUS ON FOCUS

Use restorative poses and increase your mental training as you compete. Tone down the intensity of your yoga practice even further and ramp up your awareness of the state of your breath, body, and mind.

Longer focus sessions can include breath work, gentle but deep stretches with props, and meditation. These restorative yoga sessions will keep you balanced and prepared for competition and will enhance your recovery. Slot them the afternoon of a hard or long workout or race as well as on your rest day. Following are some hour-long routines.

Focus Routine 1 (1 hr.)

Centering
The breath in space
Spinal warm-up, prone
Supported back bends
Wall folds
Inversions
Reclining twists
Corpse pose
Counting meditation
Closing

CENTERING
> p. 61

THE BREATH IN SPACE
> p. 62

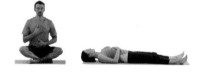

SPINAL WARM-UP, PRONE
> p. 12

SUPPORTED BACK BENDS
> p. 37

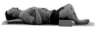
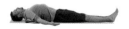

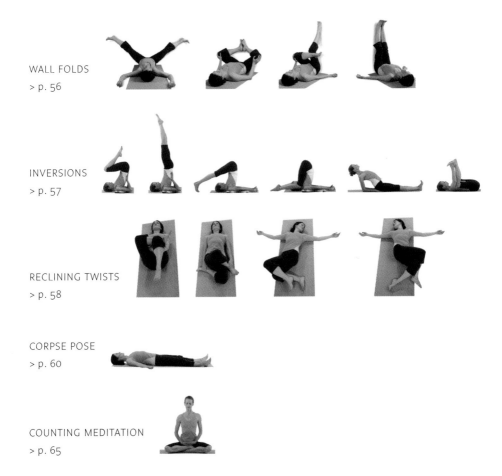

WALL FOLDS
> p. 56

INVERSIONS
> p. 57

RECLINING TWISTS
> p. 58

CORPSE POSE
> p. 60

COUNTING MEDITATION
> p. 65

CLOSING
> p. 67

Focus Routine 2 (1 hr.)

Centering
The breath in time
Spinal warm-up, supine
Gentle stretches
Corpse pose
Counting meditation
Observation meditation
Closing

CENTERING
> p. 61

  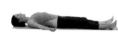

THE BREATH IN TIME
> p. 63

SPINAL WARM-UP, SUPINE
> p. 13

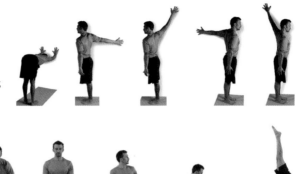

GENTLE STRETCHES
> pp. 54-55

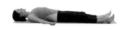

CORPSE POSE
> p. 60

COUNTING MEDITATION
> p. 65

OBSERVATION MEDITATION
> p. 66

CLOSING
> p. 67

Focus Routine 3 (1 hr.)

Centering
Counting meditation
Alternate-nostril breathing
Interlaced fingers series
Supported stretches
Corpse pose
Observation meditation
Closing

CENTERING
> p. 61

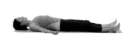

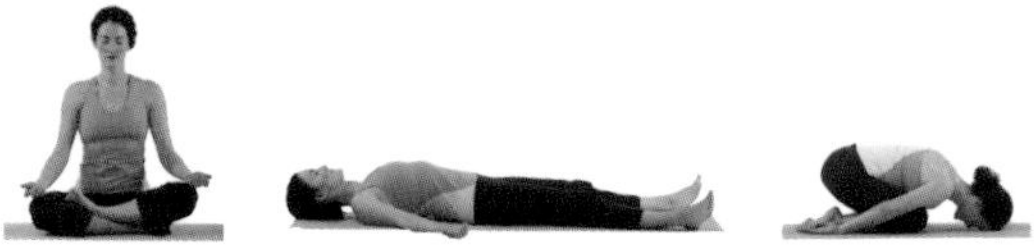

COUNTING MEDITATION
> p. 65

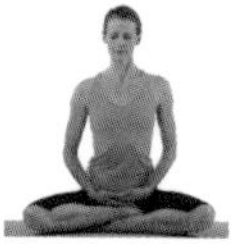

ALTERNATE-NOSTRIL BREATHING
> p. 64

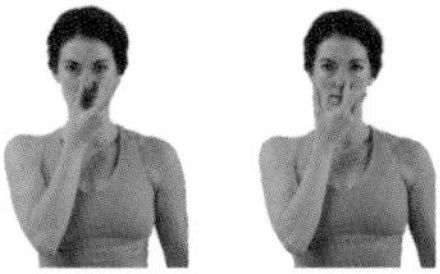

INTERLACED FINGERS SERIES
> p. 39

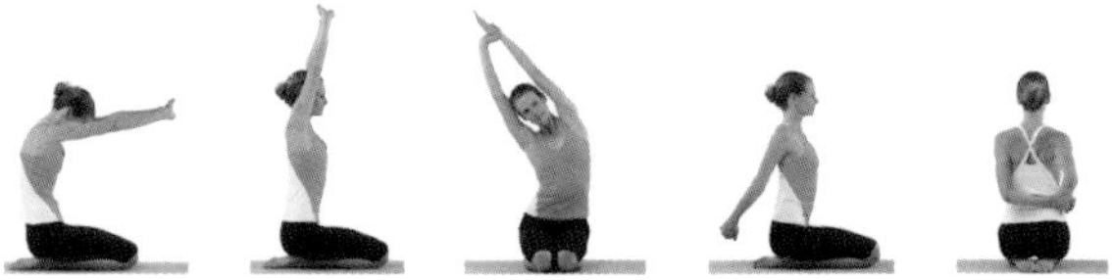

SUPPORTED STRETCHES
> p. 59

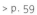

CORPSE POSE
> p. 60

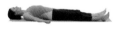

OBSERVATION MEDITATION
> p. 66

CLOSING
> p. 67

Shorter Focus Routines

These sessions might involve simply centering, a breath exercise, and meditation. Choose both the exercises and meditations you find easy and the ones you find challenging. Here are some twenty-minute combinations.

Shorter Focus Routine 1 (20 min.)

Centering
The breath in space
Counting meditation
Closing

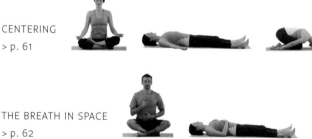

CENTERING
> p. 61

THE BREATH IN SPACE
> p. 62

COUNTING MEDITATION
> p. 65

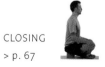

CLOSING
> p. 67

Shorter Focus Routine 2 (20 min.)

Centering
The breath in time
Observation meditation
Closing

CENTERING
> p. 61

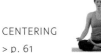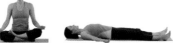

THE BREATH IN TIME
> p. 63

OBSERVATION MEDITATION
> p. 66

CLOSING
> p. 67

Shorter Focus Routine 3 (20 min.)

Centering
Alternate-nostril breathing
Counting meditation
Observation meditation
Closing

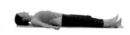

CENTERING
> p. 61

ALTERNATE-NOSTRIL BREATHING
> p. 64

COUNTING MEDITATION
> p. 65

OBSERVATION MEDITATION
> p. 66

CLOSING
> p. 67

RESOURCES

BOOKS

Baptiste, Baron. *Journey into Power: How to Sculpt Your Ideal Body, Free Your True Self, and Transform Your Life with Yoga.* New York: Fireside, 2003.

Bender Birch, Beryl. *Power Yoga: The Total Strength and Flexibility Workout.* New York: Fireside, 1995.

Couch, Jean. *The Runner's Yoga Book,* rev. ed. Berkeley, Calif.: Rodmell, 1990.

Faulds, Richard. *Kripalu Yoga: A Guide to Practice on and off the Mat.* New York: Bantam Dell, 2006.

Gunaratana, Bhante H. *Mindfulness in Plain English.* Somerville, Mass.: Wisdom, 2002.

Iyengar, B. K. S. *Light on Yoga.* New York: Schocken, 1994.

Lee, Cyndi. *Yoga Body, Buddha Mind.* New York: Riverhead, 2004.

Rountree, Sage. *The Athlete's Guide to Yoga: An Integrated Approach to Strength, Flexibility and Focus.* Boulder, Colo.: VeloPress, 2008.

Schiffmann, Erich. *Yoga: The Spirit and Practice of Moving into Stillness.* New York: Pocket, 1996.

DVDS

Dubs, Karen. *Flexible Warrior* series. Spinervals, 2007.

Grilley, Paul. *Yin Yoga.* Pranamaya, 2005.

Potter, Kate. *Namaste Yoga.* Omni Film, 2005.

Powers, Sarah. *Insight Yoga.* Pranamaya, 2005.

Rea, Shiva. *Yoga Shakti*. Gemini Sun, 2004.

Rountree, Sage. *The Athlete's Guide to Yoga: A Personalized Practice*. Endurance Films, 2008.

ONLINE RESOURCES

gaiam.com

huggermugger.com

kripalu.org

sagerountree.com

yogajournal.com

yogamatic.com

ACKNOWLEDGMENTS

Thanks to Courtney Long and Mike Forsterling for their helpful comments on the manuscript for this book. Thanks to my students and coaching clients for their explicit and implicit feedback on the benefits of yoga for athletes. Thanks to Bob Kern and to everyone at VeloPress for their continued support. Thanks to my husband, Wes, for his steadiness and steadfastness. And thanks to you for reading.

ABOUT THE MODELS

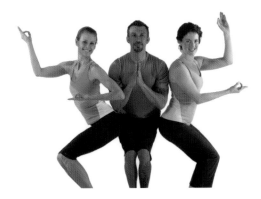

Rops Malachi Melville found her way to yoga after injuring her back as a long-distance runner. A senior teacher at Yoga Works in Los Angeles, she leads teacher training sessions and retreats worldwide. For over three years, she has been the yoga teacher for Major League Soccer team Chivas USA. Malachi has appeared on the cover of *Yoga Journal* as well as inside the magazine. Although she continues to run, it is through her yoga practice that she is pain-free and at peace.

Since his childhood on the island of Maui, **Stephen Uvalle** has enjoyed surfing, hiking, and the many experiences life affords. He is thankful for his loving child, Isabella Rose, and for all of his teachers—both the ones he enjoyed and those who agitated. He lives and teaches yoga in Boulder, Colorado.

ABOUT THE AUTHOR

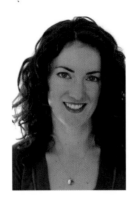

Sage Rountree is a registered yoga teacher, USA Triathlon-certified expert coach, Road Runners Club of America-certified coach, and USA Cycling coach. She holds a PhD in English and is the author of *The Athlete's Guide to Yoga* and *The Athlete's Guide to Yoga DVD,* in addition to contributing to *Runner's World* and *Yoga Journal Online.* Sage competes as an age grouper at events from the 5K to the Iron-distance triathlon, and she raced for Team USA at the 2008 Short-Course Triathlon World Championship. Her coaching clients compete in running, ultrarunning, and multisport events, including the Ironman World Championship 70.3 and both long- and short-course duathlon world championships. She teaches workshops on yoga for athletes nationwide; her schedule appears at sagerountree.com.

Sage lives in Chapel Hill, North Carolina, with her husband, Wes, and their daughters, Lily and Vivian.

sagerountree.com

ALSO AVAILABLE FROM VELOPRESS

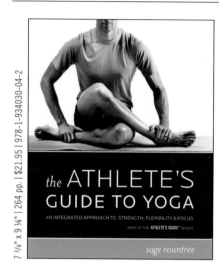

7 3/8" x 9 1/4" | 264 pp. | $21.95 | 978-1-934030-04-2

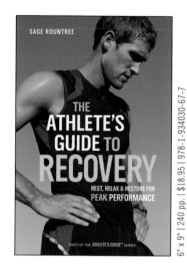

6" x 9" | 240 pp. | $18.95 | 978-1-934030-67-7

THE ATHLETE'S GUIDE TO YOGA: AN INTEGRATED APPROACH TO STRENGTH, FLEXIBILITY, AND FOCUS

Yoga makes good athletes even better by improving economy and reducing the chance of injury. In this comprehensive guide on the benefits and practice of yoga for athletes, Rountree explains how athletes should incorporate yoga into their regular training program. Full-color photographs throughout.

THE ATHLETE'S GUIDE TO RECOVERY: REST, RELAX, AND RESTORE FOR PEAK PERFORMANCE

Athletes who neglect their recovery will gain little from workouts, risking injury, overtraining, and burnout. In this book, Rountree offers the first comprehensive, practical exploration of the art and science of athletic rest. Athletes will learn how much rest they need, how to measure fatigue, and how to make the best use of recovery aids like ice baths, compression apparel, massage, and more.

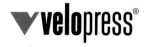